THE FAST

WAY

Heal Inflammation, Lose Weight and Have a High Functioning Body System

FERNANDEZ DAVE

Contents

INTRODUCTION 3

CHAPTER 1 4

   CHRONIC INFLAMMATION AND WEIGHT GAIN 4

      What is inflammation? 5

      What is chronic inflammation? 5

      What inflammation means for the body? 6

      How Inflammation Causes Weight Acquire ? 7

      What causes inflammation in your body? 8

      What are inflammation markers? 9

      What are inflammation causing food varieties? 9

Does dairy cause inflammation? 10

Food Varieties That Decrease Constant Inflammation 11

Diminishing Inflammation In The Body 12

Utilizing Nourishing Enhancements To Battle Inflammation 14

CHAPTER 2 16

THE ADVANTAGES OF FASTING..16

What are the advantages of fasting? 17

When do the advantages of fasting start? 18

Who profits by fasting? 19

Are there any wellbeing chances related to fasting?..............19

   Who ought to abstain from fasting? 20

How does fasting advance weight reduction? 20

Would I be able to exercise while fasting?...........................21

Can fasting diminish the danger of infection? 21

CHAPTER 3 24

PRESCRIPTIONS KNOWN TO CAUSE WEIGHT GAIN 24

What You Can Do? 28

CHAPTER 4 30

AN ANTI-INFLAMMATORY DIET: WHAT TO EAT AND WHY IT
MAKES A DIFFERENCE 30

To start with, what is inflammation? 31

When is inflammation tricky? 32

Why is persistent inflammation awful? 33

Where diet comes in? 34

Mitigating food varieties: the "short rundown".................34

CHAPTER 5 36

TOP 10 STANDARDS OF ANTI-INFLAMMATORY DIET...............36

CHAPTER 6 42

THE BEST MITIGATING FOOD SOURCES FOR WEIGHT
REDUCTION 42

CONCLUSION...50

INTRODUCTION

All in all, illnesses identified with ongoing inflammation represent half of passings around the world. The connection between stoutness, inflammation, and metabolic disorder is an interconnected web that is driving scientists to reconsider how we approach the subject of weight. Being encouraged to get thinner for wellbeing reasons is muddled in light of the fact that it regularly includes legislative issues, clinical inclination, societal position, self-perception, disgrace, and economics. Subsequently, it is additionally a medical problem that frequently isn't tended to in similar therapeutically viable and target way as other ailments.

Stoutness is connected to; coronary illness, stroke, type 2 diabetes, and certain malignancies. Weight reduction and calorie limitation have been appeared to diminish inflammation and increment insulin affectability in individuals who have been medicinally encouraged to lose abundance weight. Weight is regularly important for a troublesome cycle, however breaking this cycle isn't incomprehensible. Understanding the connection among inflammation and stoutness can likewise be a method of showing up at another way to deal with wellbeing and weight reduction.

CHAPTER 1

CHRONIC INFLAMMATION AND WEIGHT GAIN

Clinical therapies for constant infection and even weight reduction are zeroing in increasingly more on the need to forestall and diminish persistent inflammation. Studies show that inflammation is a typical basic factor taking all things together major degenerative sicknesses — including coronary illness, malignancy, hypertension, and diabetes — and that it can likewise cause weight gain and trouble shedding pounds.

The uplifting news: inflammation is connected to a few eating routine and way of life factors. By rolling out key improvements in these regions, you can lessen inflammation in the body, bring down your danger of degenerative sickness, and help your body shed overabundance weight. Keep perusing to get familiar with inflammation, what it means for your wellbeing, and how to diminish it.

What is inflammation?

Inflammation is your body's reaction to a physical issue or danger. In specific circumstances, inflammation is essential and supportive. Hitting your toe or cutting your finger can cause what's known as intense inflammation, which is portrayed by four key markers: redness, warmth, expanding, and torment. Blood stream increments to the territory so that white platelets can gather at the site of the injury and help secure the body against infection and unfamiliar trespassers, like microorganisms.

This provocative reaction is your body's method of shielding itself and fixing harmed tissue. Without intense inflammation, wounds could never recuperate. Intense inflammation is impermanent and ordinarily disappears following a couple of days.

Ongoing inflammation, then again, happens inside the body and can prompt significant unexpected issues — including weight acquire.

What is chronic inflammation?

At the point when cells are harmed within the body, a similar fiery reaction happens. Notwithstanding, constant inflammation can endure for quite a long time or years if the issue isn't dispensed with. Sometimes, inflammation can proceed regardless of whether the danger is disposed of.

Persistent inflammation, likewise alluded to as foundational inflammation, places your body into a crisis state for a delayed timeframe, which can prompt medical issues. White platelets may start assaulting sound tissue and organs, causing significantly more inflammation that can influence measures all through the body.

What inflammation means for the body?

Constant inflammation can disable capacities all through the body identified with cardiovascular wellbeing, intellectual capacity, absorption, digestion, chemical levels, and the sky is the limit from there.

At the point when fiery cells are available in the body for an all-encompassing period, it can advance the development of hazardous plaque in the courses. As plaque keeps on building, it expands the danger of coronary failure or stroke.

Also, incendiary cells in the mind may assume a part in Alzheimer's illness and dementia. Significant degrees of provocative markers have likewise been connected to sadness.

Ongoing inflammation harms the covering of the gut and can prompt flawed gut disorder, otherwise called intestinal porousness. As well as causing stomach related problems, defective gut condition permits substances from food and different sources to spill into your circulation system and cause harm to inside organs and typical real cycles.

Exploration additionally shows that inflammation is associated with tumor movement, and that numerous destructive tumors start at destinations of persistent disturbance and inflammation.

How Inflammation Causes Weight Acquire ?

Inflammation can likewise influence body weight from multiple points of view. At the point when the resistant framework identifies a danger, the body discharges substances called cytokines, which initiate the body's invulnerable reaction. Cytokines are favorable to incendiary, and they likewise meddle with the body's insulin reaction.

At the point when the body gets impervious to insulin, the pancreas should deliver a greater amount of it, which triggers the body to store fat. People with insulin obstruction will in general store more fat in the stomach area.

This stomach fat is especially risky. It expands creation of cytokines, which thus builds the danger of coronary illness. Paunch fat is likewise connected to an expanded danger of disease.

Inflammation can likewise meddle with the body's reaction to leptin, a chemical that tells the mind when you've had enough to eat. On the off chance that your mind doesn't get this sign, it can make you eat more than needed. Protection from leptin is presently thought to be a significant driver of weight acquire in people.

What causes inflammation in your body?

Anything that causes cell harm or glitch can trigger an incendiary reaction inside the body. This cell harm can be brought about by variables like openness to poisons, helpless nourishment, and bacterial irregular characteristics in the gut.

Some regular reasons for inflammation include:

•   Chronic stress. Stress prompts raised degrees of cortisol, which is additionally connected to expanded stomach fat.

•   Exposure to synthetics, including food added substances, pesticides, and ecological contamination. Skincare items and beautifying agents frequently contain phthalates, which are connected to oxidative pressure and inflammation.

- Smoking

- Nutritional inadequacies. Any supplement insufficiency can prompt cell harm either straightforwardly or in a roundabout way, yet some are particularly known to cause inflammation, including low degrees of nutrient D, nutrient B6, and nutrient B12.

- Excess weight can likewise build inflammation, as it can put weight on the body that prompts extra cell harm.

What are inflammation markers?

Persistent inflammation isn't generally clear since it is inner. Manifestations like abundance stomach weight, weakness, mouth injuries, skin issues, cerebrum mist, and joint torment might be a sign of fundamental inflammation.

Certain fiery markers can likewise be estimated with a blood test. One such marker is c-receptive protein, a substance created by the liver in light of inflammation. Exploration has discovered that men with undeniable degrees of CRP had twofold the danger of stroke and multiple times the danger of coronary episode as men with almost no inflammation.

What are inflammation causing food varieties?

Certain food sources normally trigger inflammation in the body. These incorporate sugar, vegetable oils, seared food varieties, refined starches, counterfeit sugars, and other fake food added substances.

A considerable lot of these food varieties add to the arrangement of corrosive in the body, which builds inflammation. Other corrosive shaping food varieties incorporate espresso, dairy items, pop, most games drinks, packaged natural product juice, potato chips, liquor, handled meats, and red meat.

Sugar specifically is known to drive inflammation. An investigation of 29 sound grown-ups tracked down that the individuals who burned-through only one sugar-improved refreshment each day experienced expansions in C - responsive protein and insulin opposition, just as LDL cholesterol.

Does dairy cause inflammation?

Proof on the connection between dairy items and inflammation is blended. A few examinations demonstrate that the utilization of dairy items doesn't increment fiery markers. Nonetheless, because dairy is corrosive shaping, dairy items could additionally add to an acidic inner climate, which adds to the inflammation.

Ordinary dairy items are added regularly stacked with chemicals and anti-toxins. If you will likely lessen inflammation, it could be savvy to keep away from dairy items and use options, for example, almond milk.

Food Varieties That Decrease Constant Inflammation

To battle inflammation, try including sound, entire products of the soil in each dinner. Additionally, drink a lot of water for the duration of the day to help flush poisons and waste from your body.

A few food sources offer particularly amazing anti-inflammatory benefits as cell reinforcements, nutrients, and minerals that help battle inflammation while likewise boosting your digestion.

Best food varieties for inflammation

- Leafy greens (kale, spinach)

- Green vegetables like broccoli

- Olives and olive oil

- Coconut oil

- Fatty fish (salmon, sardines, herring, mackerel)

- Berries (strawberries, blueberries, raspberries, blackberries)

- Grapes

- Cherries

- Tomatoes

- Bell peppers and stew peppers

- Mushrooms

- Avocados

- Nuts

- Seeds

- Turmeric

- Dark chocolate

- Green tea

Diminishing Inflammation In The Body

Given the wide scope of variables that add to the inflammation, obviously diminishing inflammation in the body ought to be a multi-layered methodology.

Eating a solid eating regimen brimming with mitigating food varieties is a significant advance in battling ongoing inflammation. Diminish your admission of provocative and acidic food varieties like prepared food sources, seared food varieties, and refined starches, including sugar.

It's critical to note, in any case, that changing your eating regimen alone may not be sufficient to free your group of inflammation. Conditions, for example, the broken gut disorder can keep your body from engrossing the supplements it needs from your food. Hormonal irregular characteristics, as demonstrated above, can likewise meddle with your body's reaction to food. A anti-inflammatory diet should likewise incorporate measures to help recuperate the gut and right any hormonal awkward nature.

Practices, for example, discontinuous fasting are successful in lessening inflammation and assisting with resetting the digestion so the body can work at an ideal level and better react to a solid eating regimen.

Practicing routinely and getting a lot of rest are likewise significant segments of a mitigating way of life.

To lessen your openness to synthetic compounds, use skincare items and beauty care products that are liberated from phthalates, and pick food holders and water bottles that at sans BPA. Try not to smoke, and restrict your openness to used smoke.

Likewise, receive great pressure the board methods, like care reflection. Yoga breathing activities have additionally been found to help diminish inflammation.

Utilizing Nourishing Enhancements To Battle Inflammation

Some nourishing enhancements can additionally help you battle inflammation. B nutrients can help decrease persistent inflammation, just as omega-3 unsaturated fats, calcium, magnesium, and nutrient D.

Take fish oil enhancements to close down provocative pathways, and utilize a nutrient B12 supplement to help control levels of cytokines.

CHAPTER 2

THE ADVANTAGES OF FASTING

Have you at any point had a go at fasting? Irregular fasting is an intriguing issue in the weight reduction and health networks, however, it's not without debate. Some clinical experts caution that fasting eats less is only a perilous pattern, yet the advantages of fasting have been broadly considered and are all around reported. Before beginning any sort of fasting diet, ensure you see how to do so securely, and get the endorsement of your PCP.

Fasting is the same old thing. Individuals have been fasting forever ago, regardless of whether for strict purposes or due to legitimate needs during seasons of food shortage. Presently, research is showing that this kind of way of life really had wellbeing benefits over the way we live today. These days, a significant number of us are acclimated with eating at whatever point hunger hits. We may nibble the entire day and eat late around evening time. Be that as it may, our bodies are not intended to be in this consistent condition of assimilation.

The individuals who caution against fasting frequently guarantee that this eating less junk food strategy is superfluous because our bodies have an inherent detoxification framework. This is valid, however, a large portion of us don't permit it to work appropriately. Our bodies can't process and detoxify simultaneously. At the point when we're continually eating, we keep our bodies in a steady condition of assimilation. This can prompt various medical conditions including trouble shedding pounds, stomach-related issues, weariness and laziness, joint agony, muscle throbs, migraines, rest issues, and a debilitated invulnerable framework. We frequently think about these medical problems as a characteristic piece of getting more seasoned, however, they don't need to be. Resting your stomach-related framework through occasional fasting can frequently clear up a considerable lot of these medical problems.

What are the advantages of fasting?

Fasting has been appeared to upgrade the body's protection from harming free revolutionaries that drive inflammation and help in cell fix, which can avoid malignant growth. Fasting has likewise been appeared to improve a few danger factors for coronary illness, including high LDL cholesterol, hypertension, and blood fatty substances. Improved glucose and insulin obstruction that outcomes from fasting can diminish the danger of type 2 diabetes.

Fasting offers various advantages for mental wellbeing also. Fasting can prod the development of new nerve cells, which improves mind work. It can likewise expand the creation of mind chemicals that diminish the danger of despondency. Fasting may help forestall or postpone the beginning of Alzheimer's infection, alongside neurodegenerative illnesses like Parkinson's and Huntington's sickness.

Different advantages of fasting incorporate upgraded fat consumption and muscle acquire, expanded life expectancy, and expanded energy and mental clearness.

When do the advantages of fasting start?

The impacts and advantages of fasting start promptly, however, results may not be clear until some other time. Everybody's digestion and body are interesting and will unexpectedly react to fasting.

Individuals who quick to accomplish weight reduction may lose a normal of 7 to 10 pounds inside a 10-week time frame. Your primary care physician can help you screen changes in cholesterol, circulatory strain, fatty oils, and glucose to guarantee you're encountering profits by your fasting convention.

Who profits by fasting?

Any individual who needs to improve their general wellbeing and health can profit by fasting. Individuals who may profit the most from fasting are the individuals who need to lose an abundance of weight, and who need to improve corpulence-related conditions, for example, hypertension, high glucose, and elevated cholesterol. Fasting may likewise help improve gut wellbeing in individuals who experience the ill effects of immune system problems like Crohn's infection and colitis.

Are there any wellbeing chances related to fasting?

Fasting is most secure when led under clinical watch. The individuals who are new to fasting might be in danger of parchedness on the off chance that they neglect to drink sufficient water during their fasting period. Fasting may likewise cause results, for example, cravings for food, a sleeping disorder, stress, migraine, and indigestion, yet these are commonly fleeting. In case you're keen on beginning a fasting diet to lose overabundance weight, get some information about therapeutically regulated get-healthy plans that join fasting.

Who ought to abstain from fasting?

Fasting isn't ideal for individuals who are underweight or who experience the ill effects of dietary problems like bulimia. Fasting is likewise not suggested for individuals younger than 18, individuals with type 1 diabetes, pregnant ladies, and individuals recuperating from a medical procedure.

How does fasting advance weight reduction?

It might shock no one that fasting can help advance weight reduction. Individuals frequently accept this is basically because you are eating fewer calories when fasting, however, it's, in reality, more convoluted than that. Fasting advances changes all through the body, for example, sound chemical levels and diminished inflammation, which assist the body with getting more fit all the more viably. Truth be told, contemplates show that a kind of fasting known as time-limited taking care of can help in weight reduction, in any event, when individuals burn-through a similar complete number of calories for the duration of the day.

Time-limited taking care of is the act of eating the entirety of your food inside a more limited window. For instance, eating the entirety of your dinners during an 8-hour window, for example, between 10 am and 6 pm, leaves 16 hours for your body to process and detoxify. This kind of fasting is regularly alluded to as 16/8 irregular fasting.

An investigation on the impacts of about two months of time-confined benefiting from solid guys showed a reduction in fat mass with no deficiency of bulk. Members additionally experienced expanded degrees of adiponectin, a chemical that directs measures identified with glucose usage and insulin affectability. Low degrees of adiponectin have been connected to trouble shedding pounds and a higher danger of type 2 diabetes.

Would I be able to exercise while fasting?

You can practice while fasting, yet tunes in to your body and stop in case you're feeling exhausted, frail, or weak. Time-confined taking care of can help you feel fierier in the first part of the day, which is an ideal chance to fit in your activity meeting. In case you're feeling excessively drained or lazy, skirt any focused energy exercises and take a walk or do yoga. Converse with your PCP about building up an activity routine you can adhere to while fasting.

Can fasting diminish the danger of infection?

Different sorts of fasting abstain from food have been appeared to lessen the danger of old enough related illness and may even advance cell revival. Members who finished three patterns of a fasting-mirroring diet encountered a few positive changes, including:

- A 5.9% diminishing in fasting glucose

- A 15% decrease in insulin-like development factor 1, a chemical connected to an expanded danger of malignant growth

- A 3% decrease in body weight, with a significant bit of the fat misfortune coming from stomach fat, which is connected to an expanded danger of medical issues like diabetes, stroke, coronary illness, malignancy, and even dementia

A fasting-impersonating diet additionally alluded to as "fasting with food," includes confining calories for a time of at any rate 5 days and devouring just food sources that are not difficult to process, like vegetable soup. This permits the body to go into a fasting state without totally abandoning food.

CHAPTER 3

PRESCRIPTIONS KNOWN TO CAUSE WEIGHT GAIN

Large numbers of us battle to keep a solid weight. For individuals who take certain doctor-prescribed prescriptions, additional pounds might be an undesirable result. The most well-known prescriptions that add to weight acquire are two regularly recommended drug classes—corticosteroids and antidepressants. In any case, there are others. Find out about some normal prescriptions that can prompt medication actuated weight to acquire.

Corticosteroids

Corticosteroids incorporate the anti-inflammatory drugs prednisone and hydrocortisone. Specialists recommend them to treat fiery conditions, like joint pain, dermatitis, asthma, ulcerative colitis, and Crohn's illness.

Corticosteroids can cause an increment in hunger, prompting weight to acquire. They additionally change how your body disperses fat. It will in general amass in the face, neck, back, and mid-region. This result relies upon what amount of time much and how you require for corticosteroids. Watching your eating routine and practicing can help. Any weight gain should resolve inside a couple of long periods of halting the corticosteroid.

Antidepressants

Some upper medications are more probable than others to cause weight to acquire than others. Tricyclic antidepressants, monoamine oxidase inhibitors, and serotonin reuptake inhibitors (SSRIs) will in general reason weight acquire. Its hazy how they cause it, however, their impacts on mind synthetic compounds and digestion may assume a part.

If you experience weight acquire, your primary care physician may prescribe changing to an alternate medication. There are a couple of antidepressants that are weight unbiased or that may really assist you with getting in shape. These incorporate bupropion (Wellbutrin), venlafaxine (Effexor), and duloxetine (Cymbalta).

Antipsychotic Medications

Antipsychotic medicates primarily treat bipolar confusion and schizophrenia, even though they do have different employments. Like antidepressants, some of them mess more up with weight acquire than others. Antipsychotics may cause weight to acquire through hunger incitement and indigestion changes. The trickiest ones are a portion of the second-age drugs, like clozapine (Clozaril) and olanzapine (Zyprexa). Aripiprazole (Abilify) and ziprasidone (Geodon) will in general reason fewer issues with weight acquire. Converse with your PCP to see whether one of these might work for you.

Antiseizure Medications

Specialists use antiseizure tranquilizers fundamentally to treat epilepsy and other seizure issues. Yet, this class has numerous different uses, including treating a few kinds of torment, forestalling headaches, and settling disposition. These medications influence cerebrum synthetic substances and may cause weight to acquire as a result.

Out of this gathering, carbamazepine (Tegretol), gabapentin (Neurontin), and valproic corrosive (Depakote) will in general reason the most issues. If you experience weight acquire, your PCP may suggest exchanging drugs. Lamotrigine (Lamictal), topiramate (Topamax), and zonisamide (Zonegran) might be choices.

Diabetes Medications

Some diabetes medicines can cause weight to acquire. Furthermore, everything comes down to insulin—the chemical that is missing or not working right in diabetes. Insulin advances weight acquire by controlling how your body uses and stores energy. Beginning insulin treatment frequently prompts weight to acquire. However, the medical advantages of controlling glucose levels far exceed this result. Also, working with your eating routine and exercise propensities can help oversee it.

Other diabetes medicines can cause weight to acquire by animating your body to deliver insulin. This incorporates the sulfonylureas, like glipizide (Glucotrol), and the thiazolidinediones, for example, pioglitazone (Actos).

More Medications

There are more medications and classes of medications that can cause weight to acquire. A few models incorporate beta-blockers for hypertension, antihistamines, and anti-conception medication pills. On the off chance that you are worried about weight to acquire, converse with your PCP before you start any new medication.

What's more, inform your PCP regarding any new or abnormal side affects you experience after beginning medication. Your primary care physician can decide if the medication may be the issue. Provided that this is true, you can work out an arrangement for managing the result or attempting another treatment.

What You Can Do?

In case you're ingesting doctor-prescribed medications that cause weight to acquire, you can in any case-control the numbers on your washroom scale. Your PCP may propose you make diet and way of life acclimations to try not to put on weight. Watching your supper parcels and getting sufficient normal exercise may help. On the off chance that your condition makes it hard for you to stay with diet and exercise, talk with your PCP about alternate approaches to evade medicine-related weight acquire. Techniques, for example, psychological conduct treatment or changing to an alternate sort of medicine may help.

CHAPTER 4

AN ANTI-INFLAMMATORY DIET: WHAT TO EAT AND WHY IT MAKES A DIFFERENCE

We may consider inflammation the limited growth that happens to a turned lower leg or skeletal muscles after an extraordinary exercise. In any case, there's another sort of inflammation that can immensely affect you and your customers: the sort of ongoing, foundational inflammation related to a large number of ailments and sicknesses.

You may have heard that this sort of inflammation—a side-effect of constant physical or mental pressure—can be controlled with work out. Late examination shows that moderate treadmill practice helps insusceptible cells' creation of mixtures that manage both neighborhood and foundational inflammation. Truth be told, in just 20 minutes, researchers saw changes in inflammation biomarkers.

By and large, corresponding dietary changes can upgrade the advantages of activity and, on account of inflammation, give an extra way to forestall or turn around it.

While there isn't really one "mitigating diet" to be followed, there are many prescribed procedures that are genuinely simple to utilize.

To start with, what is inflammation?

Inflammation is a fundamental normal reaction inside the human resistant framework. The insusceptible framework's job is to restrict actual harm from ailment or injury by perceiving and reacting to threats like infections, microorganisms, poisons, and surprisingly unfamiliar bodies like a splinter. For instance, when the safe framework detects a prompt danger—like a chilly infection or cell harm from a cut—it triggers something many refer to as an incendiary reaction. The reason for this reaction is to animate the influenced cells to deliver synthetic heroes, like histamines and prostaglandins, to secure against interlopers while drawing in white platelets and their contamination battling antibodies.

These cycles assume a critical part in injury mending and are valuable systems for annihilating attacking microorganisms). Calling these aides to the scene makes liquid break from the circulation system into the encompassing tissues. The resultant growing—otherwise known as inflammation—contains harm, such as enveloping a flimsy item by bubble wrap.

On account of competitors, this provocative reaction can likewise go with work out incited harm to skeletal muscle tissue brought about by an extraordinary. This doesn't imply that activity is terrible, however, it implies that inflammation can really be both acceptable and awful for you.

When is inflammation tricky?

In some cases, the resistant framework triggers an incendiary reaction to something that is definitely not a genuine danger. For instance, individuals with hypersensitivities have a fierce tempest going on inside their bodies, with their safe framework assaulting substances like pet dander, residue, and dust. In individuals with immune system illnesses, which incorporate a few sorts of joint pain, the resistant reaction is aimed at sound body cells, irritating. Inflammation can likewise be a response to persistent pressure, which restrains the chemicals that typically stifle safe reactions. This is similar to opening the conduits of a dam.

While the incendiary reaction is essential when the body needs to address a prompt concern (injury or contamination), medical issues can emerge when inflammation doesn't decrease. Persistent inflammation has been connected to the beginning and movement of numerous sorts of sicknesses, including diabetes, malignant growth, cardiovascular infections, joint pain, fiery gut illness, and weight.

Why is persistent inflammation awful?

During seasons of persistent pressure, there is expanded energy interest on the body, bringing about a higher take-up of respiratory oxygen or a "respiratory burst." To manage it, the body creates "free revolutionaries" called receptive oxygen species (ROS).

As a boost: A free extremist is a particle that is temperamental on account of an electron shortfall in its external orbital layer. Looking for security, the free extreme will interface up to another atom close by to "get" an electron. This can begin a course of harm as the "assaulted" particle (having lost an electron) presently turns into a free extreme itself and looks to glom onto one more atom. The resultant chain response can prompt harm taking all things together pieces of the influenced cell and, in the long run, cell demise. This arrangement of occasions additionally causes inflammation as the body endeavors to manage the assault.

Be that as it may, it doesn't end there: While free extremists trigger inflammation, inflammation can similarly trigger the body's creation of free revolutionaries, explicitly ROS. This - endless loop of persistent inflammation lays the right foundation for constant illness. By lessening inflammation, in any case, we can diminish oxidation—and the other way around.

Where diet comes in?

The words "oxygen" and "oxidation" carry us to the subject of cancer prevention agents. Cell reinforcements are intensified that can forestall tissue harm (counting inflammation) by connecting up with, obliterating, or forestalling the age of free extremists. The specific instruments behind this are not totally perceived. Cell reinforcements may dull the impacts of a safe reaction, cut off inflammation pathways or cycles in play during the reaction, or keep the inflammation from happening in any case.

Uplifting news: The very sort of diet that assists improve with practicing execution, weight support, and long haul wellbeing ought to likewise normally bring down inflammation.

Mitigating food varieties: the "short rundown"

There is no wizardry slug or one sorcery superfood; in any case, these are a portion of the entire food sources that have solid mitigating properties:

- Berries

- Cacao

- Citrus organic products

- Ginger

- grass-took care of meat

- Green verdant vegetables

- Green tea

- Wild-got fish

The most ideal approach to acquire the important nutrients and minerals to battle inflammation is to carry out an entire food variety diet that contains food varieties wealthy in phytochemicals—cell reinforcement supplement intensifies that have been found to have an anti-inflammatory impact. Since various food sources contain various sorts of mitigating specialists, eating a scope of food varieties with anti-inflammatory properties is the best procedure.

Much of the time, the supplements in anti-inflammatory food sources may work by shortcircuiting the incendiary reaction, restricting with free revolutionaries, and blunting the creation of the body's synthetics that trigger and add to inflammation.

CHAPTER 5

TOP 10 STANDARDS OF ANTI-INFLAMMATORY DIET

To forestall or ease inflammation, it is ideal to restrict wellsprings of unfortunate and additionally trigger food varieties and increment admission of sound, entire, common, and natural food varieties. Here are some particular prescribed procedures and tips concerning what to eat (and keep away from) to forestall or ease inflammation in the body.

1. Burn-Through In Any Event 25 Grams Of Fiber Every Day

To get your fill of fiber, search out entire grains, organic products, and vegetables. A fiber-rich eating routine decreases inflammation by providing normally happening anti-inflammatory phyto-nutrients found in organic products, vegetables, and other entire food varieties. The examination has tracked down a backward connection between biomarkers of fundamental inflammation and fiber admission: as such, the more, the better.

2. Eat a Lot of Leafy Foods

To support your admission of mitigating cell reinforcements, burn-through at any rate seven servings of vegetables and two servings of organic product consistently. One "serving" likens to a large portion of a cup of organic product or cooked vegetables or one cup of crude verdant vegetables.

Information propose that the biomarkers of inflammation influenced by entire grains are not quite the same as those influenced by foods grown from the ground, so it's imperative to burn-through both

What's more, did you realize that diets based on plants can notedly speed up weight reduction?

3. Eat Four Servings of Alliums and Crucifers Week By Week

Alliums incorporate garlic, scallions, onions, and leeks, while crucifers allude to vegetables like broccoli, cabbage, cauliflower, mustard greens, and Brussels sprouts. Alliums and crucifers contain incredible cancer prevention agent properties, so make certain to mesh them into your day-by-day produce consumption—to the tune of four servings of each week.

Exploration shows that garlic, for example, contains sulfur compounds (counting allicin) that have anti-inflammatory properties. In onions, a compound called quercetin controls. Crucifers, since quite a while ago elevated to forestall constant illness, contain isothiocyanates and indoles—particles found to diminish inflammation and oxidative pressure.

4. Burn-through OMEGA-3 Unsaturated fats

Expect to eat loads of food sources high in omega-3 unsaturated fats. Models incorporate fish, flax supper, and pecans. For individuals who are veggie lovers or veggie lovers or who don't burn-through fish, taking a decent quality vegetarian omega-3 enhancement can be useful.

Examination shows that omega-3 unsaturated fats diminish inflammation and may help bring down the danger of ongoing sicknesses like coronary illness, malignant growth, and joint pain—conditions that frequently have a high-inflammation measure at their root. Discoveries additionally recommend omega-3s to help decrease the requirement for corticosteroid meds in individuals with rheumatoid joint inflammation.

5. Trade in Unsaturated Fats

Unsaturated fats come principally from vegetables, nuts, and seeds. They contrast from immersed fats by having fewer hydrogen particles attached to their carbon chains. An examination in The American Diary of Clinical Sustenance found that individuals who ate more nuts week by week had lower inflam¬matory biomarkers.

6. Cook with Spices and Flavors

Numerous spices and flavors are known for their anti-inflammatory properties. These incorporate stew peppers, cloves, cinnamon, turmeric, ginger, rosemary, sage, and thyme.

For instance, considers have shown that enhancing with curcumin, the dynamic fixing in turmeric can help altogether improve provocative conditions like ulcerative colitis and rheumatoid joint pain. Capsaicin, a substance in stew peppers, has likewise been found to capture fiery pathways.

7. Evade Hyperpalatables

Hyperpalatables are handled food sources, refined sugars, and refined carbs that by and large contain unreasonable sugar, salt, as well as fat. This incorporates any food that contains high-fructose corn syrup or is high in sodium—the two of which add to inflammation all through the body. Sugar can initiate compound signals that instigate incendiary pathways.

8. Cutoff Soaked Fats

Immersed fats are fundamentally found in creature items; nonetheless, they are additionally found in tropical fat sources, for example, palm oil and coconut oil. Cutoff immersed fat to around 10% of everyday fat admission.

One simple technique is to pick protein sources that are lower in soaked fat, like lean meat, poultry, and fish. A few examinations have shown that immersed fats make fat tissue inflammation that can add to coronary illness and worsen generally speaking inflammation.

9. Cut out Trans Fats

In 2006, the FDA required food producers to recognize trans fats on sustenance marks—and in light of current circumstances: Studies show that individuals who eat food varieties high in trans fats have more elevated levels of C-responsive protein, a biomarker for inflammation in the body.

10. Avoid Individual Fiery Triggers

A few groups have extra ¬inflammatory issues or sensitivities. Here are few of the most widely recognized:

Gluten. In individuals with gluten affectability or celiac illness, gluten proteins are deciphered as a danger to the body. This dispatches an insusceptible reaction that assaults the digestion tracts, causes malabsorption of supplements, and can prompt auto-invulnerable problems whenever left untreated. Dairy and casein.

Devouring cow's milk may add to inflammation in your body on the off chance that you are touchy or oversensitive to lactose. Liquor. Liquor is known to add to numerous sicknesses and issues, some of which are inflammation-based.

CHAPTER 6

THE BEST MITIGATING FOOD SOURCES FOR WEIGHT REDUCTION

Diminishing inflammation can be as critical to weight reduction as diet and movement. These food sources carry out twofold responsibility with regards to decreasing inflammation and getting thinner.

Putting on weight, or the failure to shed abundance pounds is regularly a warning that there is basic second rate inflammation in the body. Also, on the other side, even the most focused eating and exercise propensities are regularly insufficient when inflammation is available. While the dynamic among weight and inflammation is perplexing, research highlights diminishing inflammation as being as fundamental to weight reduction as diet and action. So what are the best twofold obligation food sources, the ones that lessen inflammation while additionally supporting weight reduction? Here the 10 top mitigating food sources for weight reduction.

Cauliflower or broccoli "rice"

While entire grains like earthy colored rice and entire wheat pasta have a lot of advantages with regards to weight reduction (to be specific loads of useful for-you fiber), trading out carb-rich food sources like pasta and rice for riced cauliflower or broccoli can help cut calories and carbs and help mitigate inflammation. At the point when finely cleaved, these two low-carb veggies give a grain-like base to smooth or sassy dishes or can be sautéed with different veggies to incredible a low-carb pan sear. Furthermore, because cauliflower and broccoli are important for the cruciferous vegetable family, they contain different plant intensities that may have amazing mitigating impacts when eaten routinely.

Berries

Berries like strawberries and blueberries are probably the best organic product picks when attempting to get thinner, since they're low in calories and high in filling fiber. Indeed, 1 cup of cut strawberries has only 55 calories and contains 3 grams of fiber. This fiber gives a sensation of totality, and it likewise implies berries will in general have a lower glycemic reaction contrasted with numerous different organic products, which is useful for glucose the board, yearnings, and inflammation. Another advantage is their powerful portion of cancer prevention agents and anthocyanins, which assist the pack with bringing down existing and future inflammation.

Pecans

Eating a mix of fiber, protein, and sound fat at dinners and tidbits is a distinct advantage when consuming fewer calories due to the satiety this combo gives. Furthermore, tree nuts like pecans, almonds, and pistachios have an ideal equilibrium of each of the three supplements, including some mitigating omega-3 fats. While the fat and calories in nuts can add up rapidly, research recommends that people who eat around 1 ounce of nuts (around 1/4 cup) on most days are bound to be at solid body loads and more averse to put on weight, which means nuts can be an extraordinary bite, particularly in case you're attempting to get thinner. The stunt is keeping steady over divide size.

Greek yogurt

Great microbes assume a part in the processing of fiber and unsaturated fats. Along these lines, research recommends that one's gut wellbeing may affect how proficient a body is at shedding abundance weight. Besides, having a different inventory of good microorganisms is additionally useful with regards to lessening fiery mixtures that can prompt insulin opposition and weight acquire. This implies reinforcing the gut's organism obstruction is key for by and large wellbeing and body weight. Perhaps the most ideal approach to do this is to burn-through yogurt with live microscopic organisms' societies routinely. Pick Greek yogurt for more significant levels of protein (and select plain rather than seasoned to evade added sugars). At that point add a new natural product or nuts for a little pleasantness and crunch.

Beans

High-fiber beans and vegetables like dark beans, naval force beans, chickpeas, peas, and lentils are acceptable wellsprings of both protein and moderate processing starches. This mix offers transient advantages by leaving the stomach full and forestalling unexpected glucose spikes and seems to have long-haul weight reduction benefits. A recent report found that people who ate beans and vegetables most days shed pounds at a marginally higher rate than health food nuts who didn't devour beans consistently. Furthermore, from a mitigating viewpoint, beans and vegetables are ideal wellsprings of complex carbs, particularly when eaten instead of refined grains and prepared starches.

Verdant greens

Eating less junk food shouldn't leave you feeling vacant, and stacking up on non-dull vegetables like verdant greens is a decent method to add more food to your plate without adding numerous calories or carbs. Intend to start adding a small bunch or two of verdant greens like child spinach, kale, arugula, lettuces, and different greens to your plate all things considered suppers, regardless of whether it's as a plate of mixed greens or blended in with different fixings. A 2-cup serving of green like child spinach has only 27 calories and gives 3 grams of fiber, 3 mg of iron, and practically 50% of your day by day needs for nutrients An and C. What's more, regarding long haul wellbeing, verdant greens show the absolute most grounded research-supported wellbeing possibilities with regards to diminishing inflammation.

Avocado

Fat is a vital supplement required in the eating routine, however, sorting out some way to join oils and sound fats when eating fewer carbs can be somewhat overwhelming. In case you're in this boat, think about the avocado. In addition to the fact that this is a smooth natural product loaded with monounsaturated fats, nutrient E, fiber, and carotenoids which on the whole work together to relieve inflammation in the body, yet research recommends that individuals who eat avocado day by day will, in general, have lower body loads and lower BMIs. These genuinely huge outcomes were in contrast with the individuals who once in a while ate avocado or had considerably less regular utilization.

Extra-virgin olive oil

Piggy-support on the avocado, another great decision for getting those sound fats in is to pick extra-virgin olive oil. All fats and oils have around similar calories and fat per tablespoon however olive oil is a decent wellspring of those better-unsaturated fats and contains an extraordinary compound called oleocanthal which has mitigating consequences for the body. All olive oils contain oleocanthal, however, less-refined sorts like extra-virgin have more elevated levels, so make that you're go-to for a plate of mixed greens dressings and when cooking at lower warms.

Garlic and flavors

It's not difficult to stay with good dieting when you love the food you're eating, so don't be reluctant to siphon up the flavor, just as attempt new flavors. By consolidating garlic and flavors like turmeric, rosemary, cinnamon, cumin, and ginger you'll forestall feast weariness, just as quiet inflammation. While fragrant flavors and impactful garlic may seem like they can irritate inflammation, research recommends they really do the inverse. Indeed, their fragrant mixtures have been utilized restoratively in different societies for quite a long time for anti-inflammatory impacts.

Citrus natural product

A delicious citrus organic product like oranges, tangerines, and grapefruit are loaded with dissolvable fiber, settling on them a decent decision when consuming fewer calories for satiety and their low glycemic sway. Picking fiber-rich food sources like citrus may likewise offer some extra weight reduction advantages with regards to rest. Exploration proposes that eating a low-fiber diet is related to diminished rest quality. This is significant because lacking rest triggers changes that can diminish insulin affectability and increment craving and danger of weight acquire. So getting a serving of citrus every day is a low-calorie approach to get more fiber, just as a burden upon nutrient C, which is a cell reinforcement that forestalls inflammation.

CONCLUSION

In corpulent and overweight subjects weight reduction, initiated both by energy-limited eating routine or medical procedure, is a determinant factor for lessening the degree of favorable to fiery markers. Hypocaloric diet has a mitigating impact free of the eating routine organization which can assume a significant part in the avoidance of ongoing illnesses.

A propensity once educated – positive or negative – stays with us until the finish of our lives.

Self-announced specialists on changing propensities say something different and convince us that a difference in propensity is so basic, easy, and lovely, and most take one minute. All things considered, in these furious occasions, nobody possesses any energy for anything.

'Five straightforward approaches to transform unfortunate propensities into great ones'...

'To make another propensity last and cause it to supplant the one we need to change, it's sufficient to rehash it multiple times, and so forth

Also, doesn't work? That is nothing unexpected… It's no so basic. For what reason is it so difficult for us to at any rate eat good food?

A difference in propensity is an interaction and hence most importantly, needs to proceed. Additionally, it needs from you – it truly accomplishes – work, time, and space. If you have 1,000 things at the forefront of your thoughts when you don't have the opportunity to consider what you're eating regimen ought to be. You need to make room in your life for this change. Neither will you get familiar with another dialect discussing it –, in actuality, truly, you need time to learn something consistently.

Learning all alone will not give anything either, for, if you don't utilize it, you'll fail to remember it.

It's the equivalent with new propensities – on the off chance that you don't keep on debilitating old propensities and reinforce new ones so they become part of your daily schedule. At that point, even good motives when something unpleasant occurs in your life or when you're extremely drained, won't help and you will return to the old propensity.

It so happens that we are additionally the cause of all our own problems

"Examination shows that individuals who think they have the most resolve are really the destined to let completely go when enticed. For instance, smokers who are the most hopeful about their capacity to oppose allurement are well on the way to backslide four months after the fact, and over-optimistic health food nuts are the to the least extent liable to get more fit."

It merits taking work on new propensities

"Lower the initiation energy for propensities you need to embrace, and raise it for propensities you need to keep away from. The more we can lower or even dispense with the actuation energy for our ideal activities, the more we upgrade our capacity to kick off certain change."

"We shouldn't be told something so self-evident, however surely babies aren't the solitary ones who oppose truly necessary rests. Grown-ups regularly dupe themselves on rest, and the outcome is less restraint."

Brain science likewise reveals to us that on the off chance that you don't completely disallow yourself something, yet say that you'll do it later – regularly later you'll basically lose the longing. This is additionally the situation with slims down.

"... Individuals who had advised themselves "Not currently, but rather later" were less bothered with dreams of chocolate cake than the other two gatherings... Those in the deferment condition really ate essentially not exactly those in the abstinence condition... "

No change will be a triumph if you don't start by tolerating yourself as of now before presenting changes – this aids on occasion when you do not have the solidarity to deal with your changes.

"Many more than one investigation shows that self-analysis is reliably connected with less inspiration and more terrible discretion. It is likewise one of the single greatest indicators of sadness, which channels both "I will" force and "I need" power. Conversely, self-empathy—being strong and kind to yourself, particularly notwithstanding stress and disappointment—is related with more inspiration and better poise."

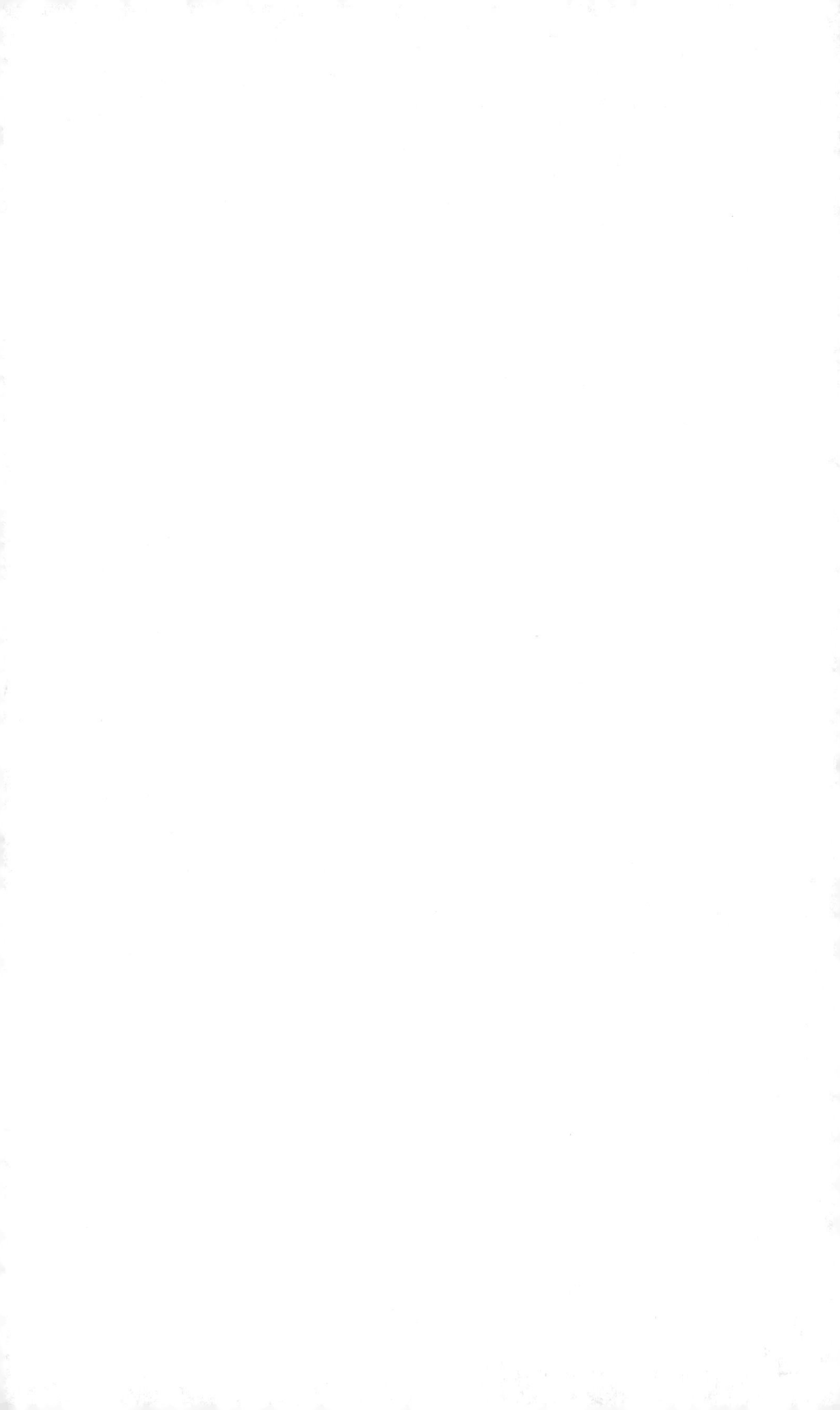